A Safe Place

A WALK WITH SELF DISCOVERY

Grounding and mediative activities to support finding your own safe space.

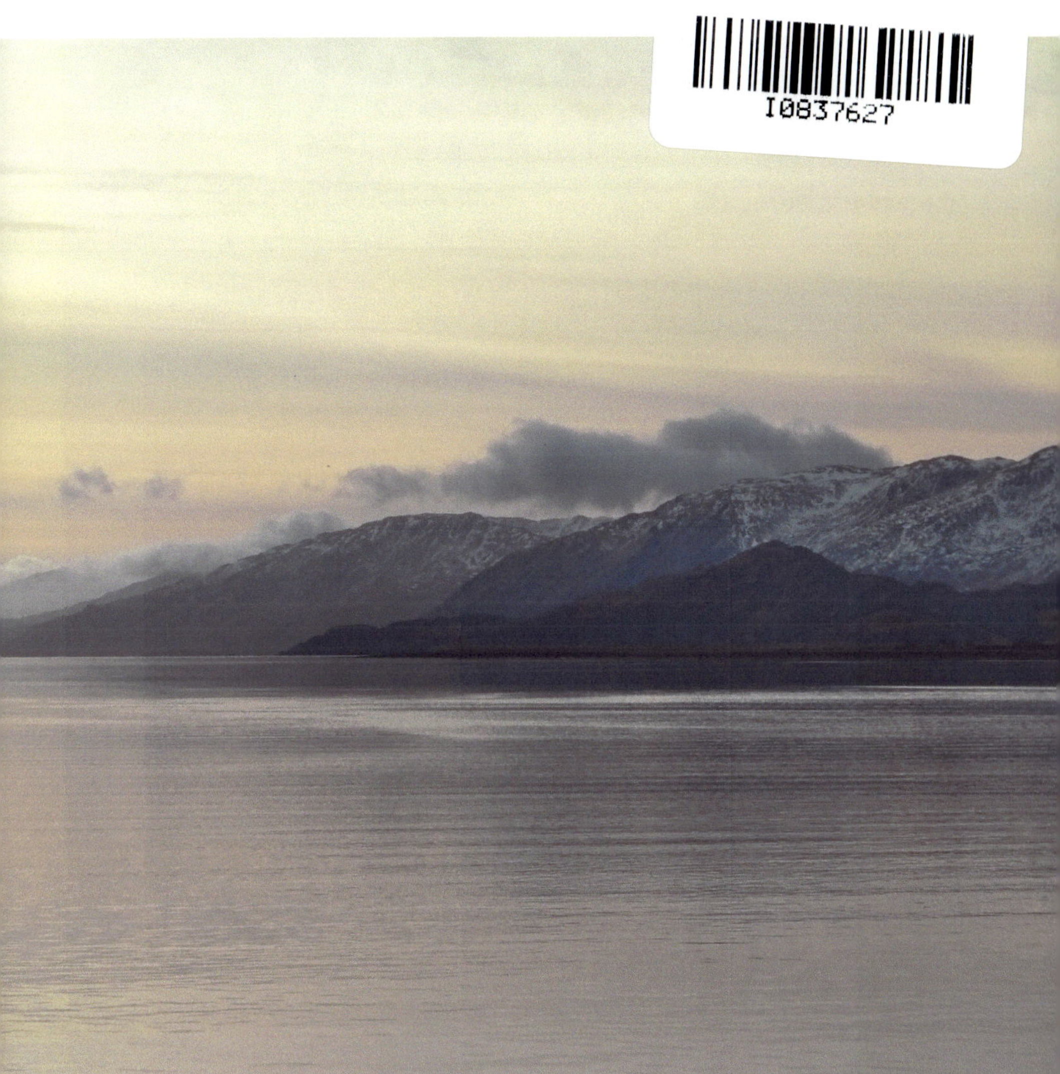

Safe Place Imagery For Wellbeing

Our brains can sometimes be intricate and cause us issues, this could be the effects of every day life, trauma, elevated stress or even just an active imagination that you find difficult to switch off. Safe place image therapy is a standard exercise for trauma therapy, but it can help you refocus and feel calmer in every day life, finding a safe place and supporting you to feel calmer and help retrain your brain and take a step back and regain a sense of peace and calm.

Feeling safe is integral to being a human, and this is not always the world we live in today. Life is busy, life can drag our emotions down and we can find ourselves on edge or anxious.

This book is full of imagery to help support you on this journey. It walks you through using safe place imagery and, through guided prompts, delves into working on the aspects the image that support a feeling of wellbeing and calmness and brining back a sense of equilibrium to your mind, body and soul. Before you start, go to a place that is comfortable to you, this could be sitting, standing, lying down, it could be out in nature, or at the park watching your children play. Take this book, a pen, and any other materials that you see fit.

The process

1. Relax, shoulders back, open your chest fully and breathe slowly, purposefully and rhythmic, then smile gently.
2. Once you feel settled, choose any 'Safe place image' in this book and look at it for a minute or two, taking in the scene and appreciating it. You may go to a few different images before you settle on one that feels right for you today, and that's fine. If in doing this you feel your mindset losing its relaxation state, return to step one and repeat.
3. Look at the image and identify what it is, what your thought processes are, what colours, shapes and sounds are present at forefront of your thought process as a result of the imagery.
4. Engage fully with the image for the whole minute or two and allow your feelings and emotions to respond to the image.
5. Slowly, allow yourself to re-ground, move your toes, logs, torso, arms, head and slowly bring focus back to your surroundings.
6. Now become reflective and work through the guided prompts on each image to further investigate your 'Safe place image'. There is a wheel of emotions in the appendix of this books to help you choose words to support your emotions, feeling and sensations.
7. Return to the book as a reflective tool at times when you feel you need a sense of calm, wellbeing and grounding brought back into your life.

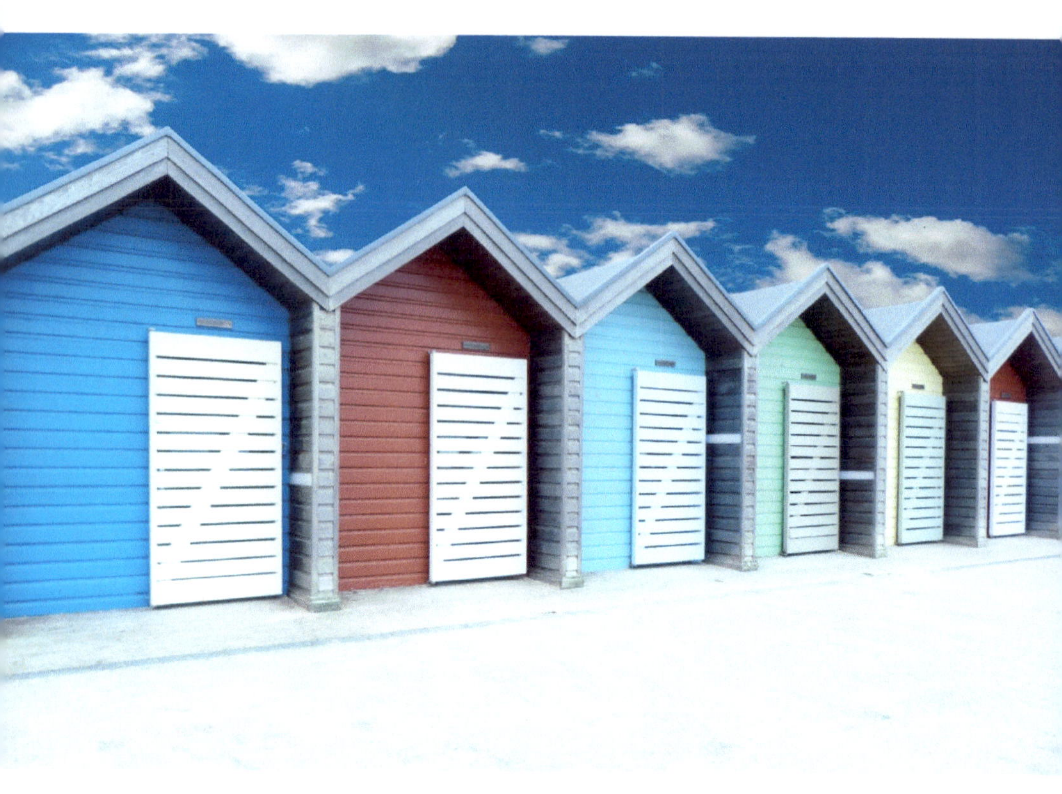

Breathe, smile, relax. What does the image make you think about?

____

____

Using the image as a focus, close your eyes, and look around, what do you see?

____

____

What can you hear?

____

____

Imagining turning from the image, what do you see?

____

____

Additional thought processes:

____

____

____

____

____

____

____

____

____

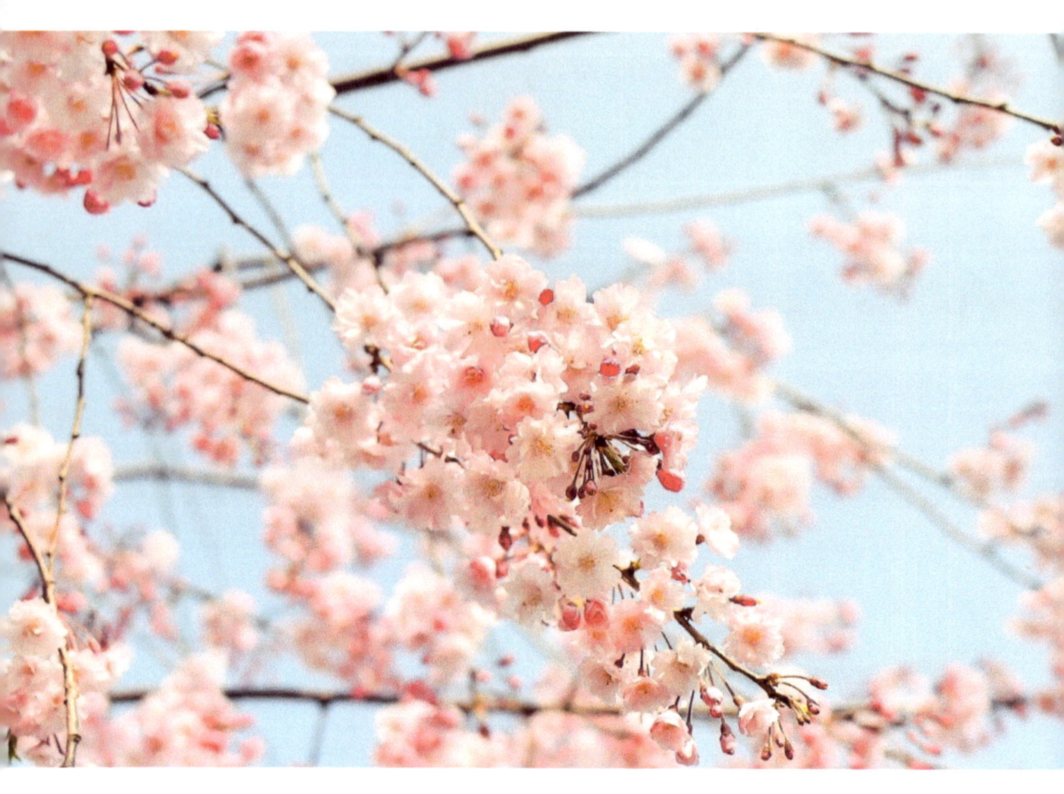

Take time to breathe slowly and purposefully, with closed eyes. Open again and describe your first feeling or emotion.

____

____

What sounds do you hear?

____

____

What scents does the image bring to mind?

____

____

Think of the colours in the image, what do they make you think about?

Additional thought processes:

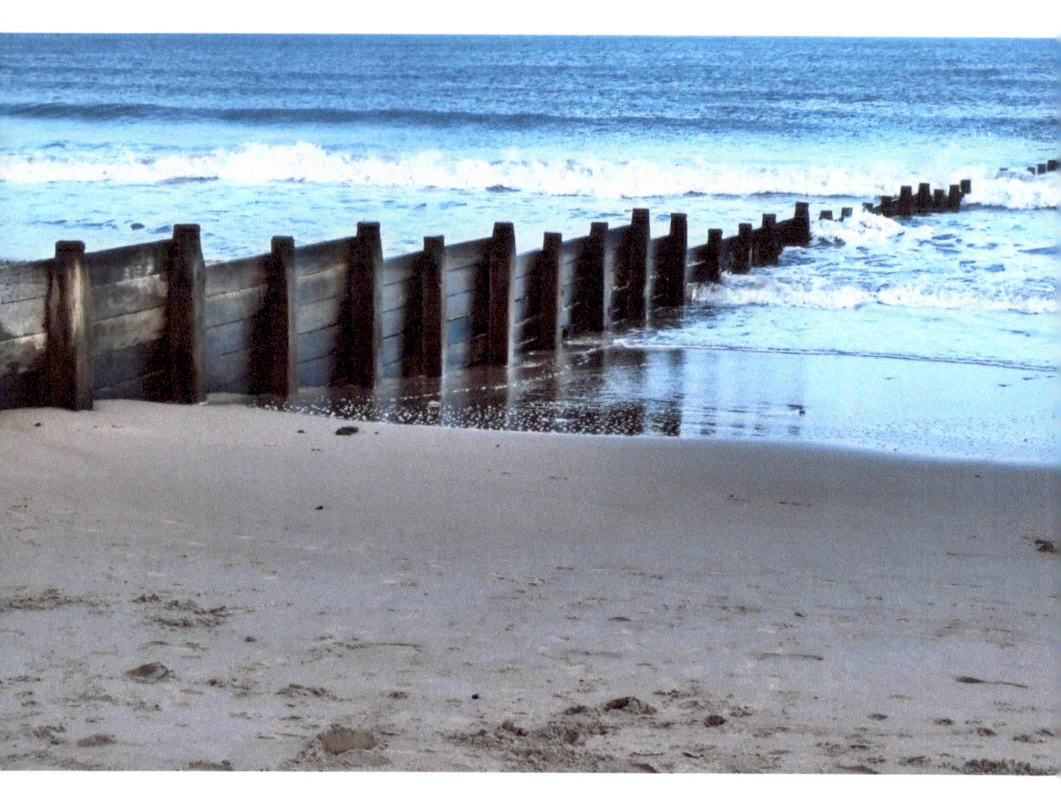

Imagine you are here, your feet are on the sand, how does that feel to you?

____

____

Close your eyes, what elements of nature do you sense?

____

____

What sensations are running through your mind as you look at this picture?

____

____

What memories does this image evoke?

____

____

Additional thought processes:

____

____

____

____

____

____

____

____

____

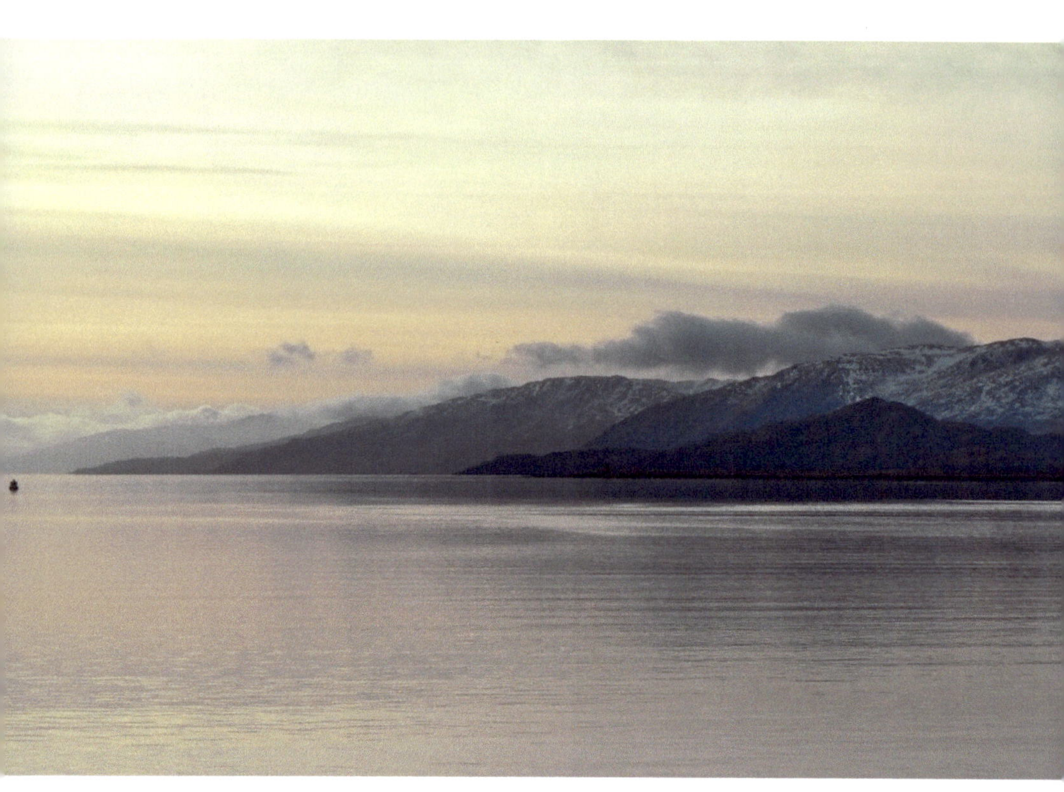

Look out to the colours in the landscape scene, what do they evoke in you?

____

____

Where do you imagine this to be?

____

____

Focus on the sensations this image is giving you; your skin, your face, movement around you?

____

____

What sensation do you feel within you?

____

____

Additional thought processes:

____

____

____

____

____

____

____

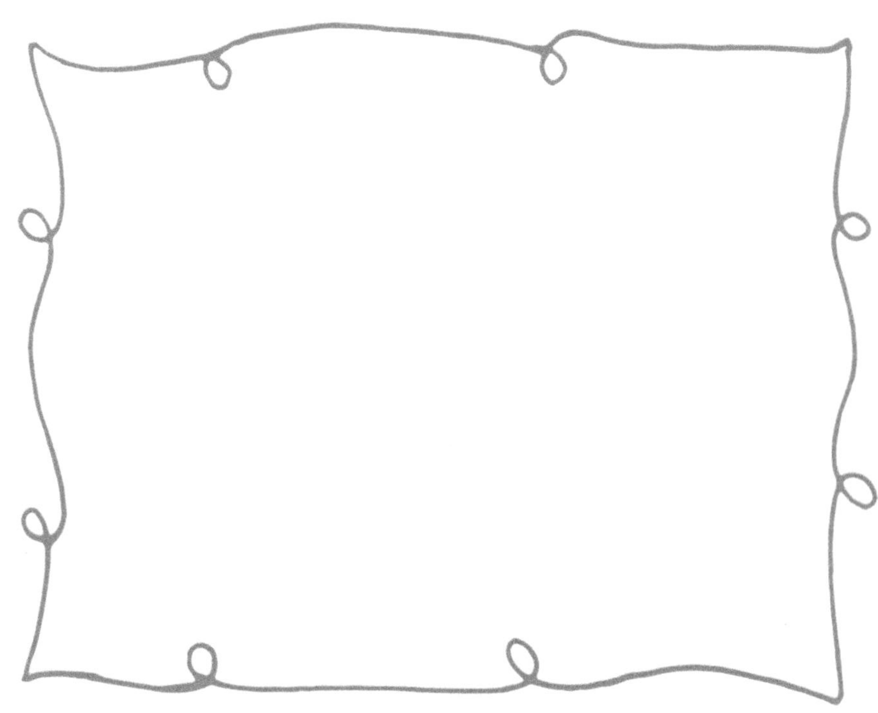

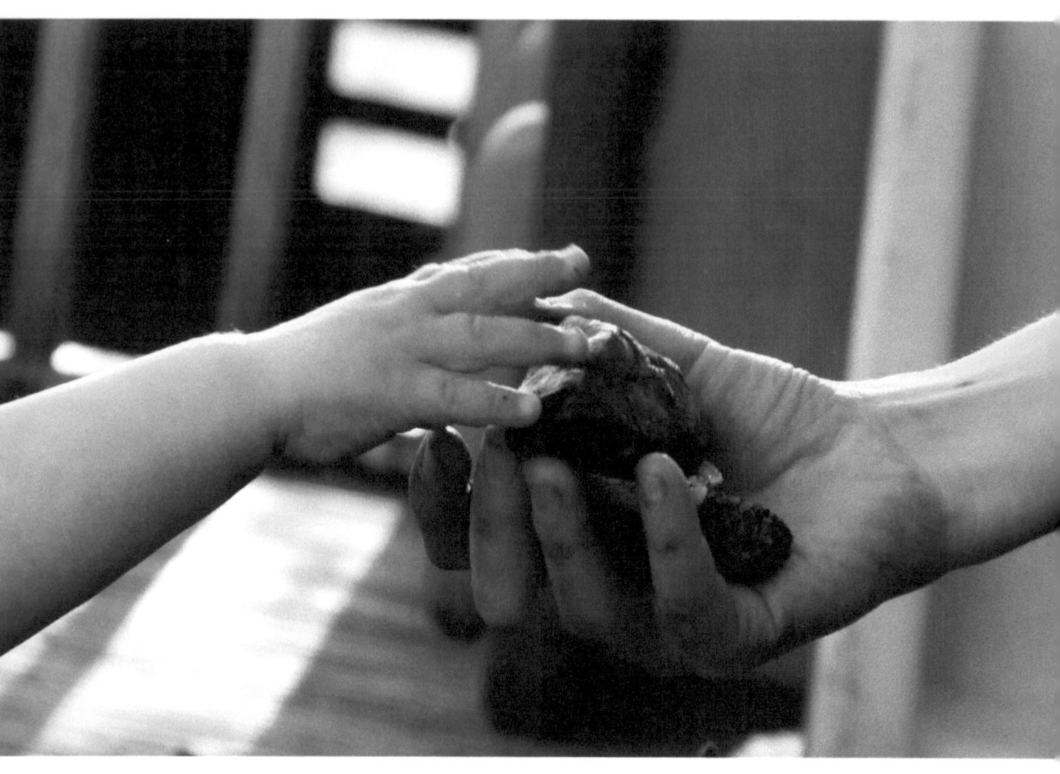

What gestures does this image give you a sense of?

____

____

What is the most noticeable sound to sense from this image?

____

____

Chose a title for this image.

____

____

Explain the reasoning behind your title choice?

____

____

Additional thought processes:

____

____

____

____

____

____

____

____

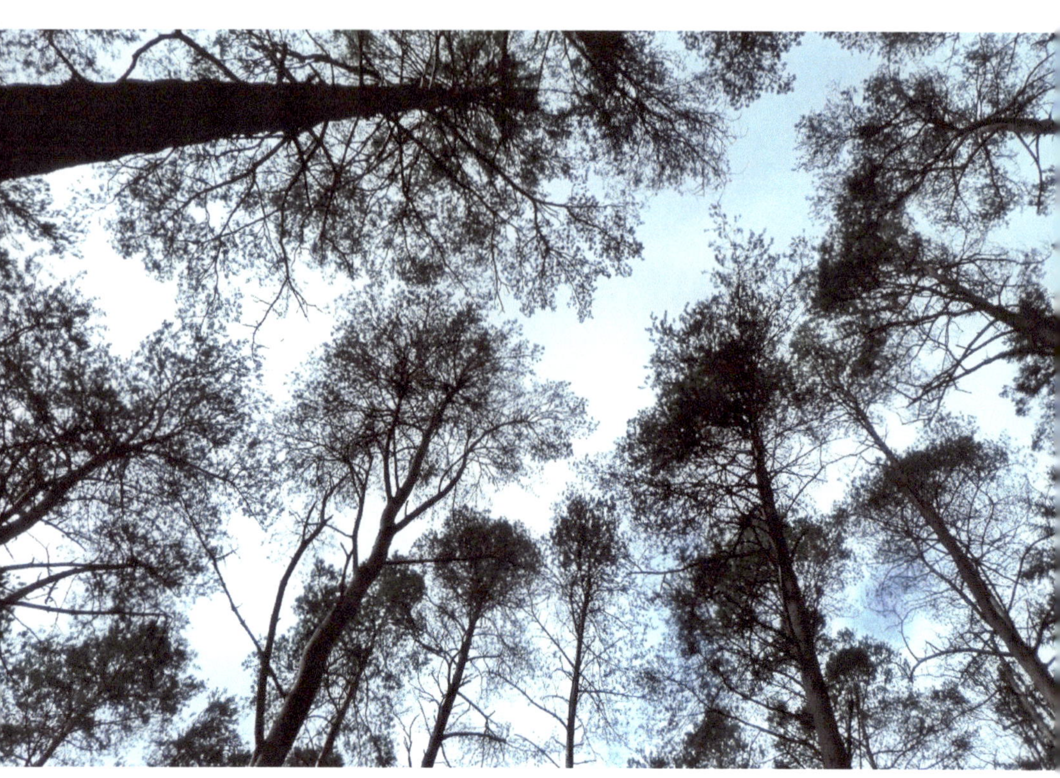

Imagine you are lying down, how do you feel looking up?

____

____

Are you hearing silence or noise?

____

____

What is below you?

____

____

Returning yourself to eye level with this image in mind, what comes to mind?

____

____

Additional thought processes:

____

____

____

____

____

____

____

____

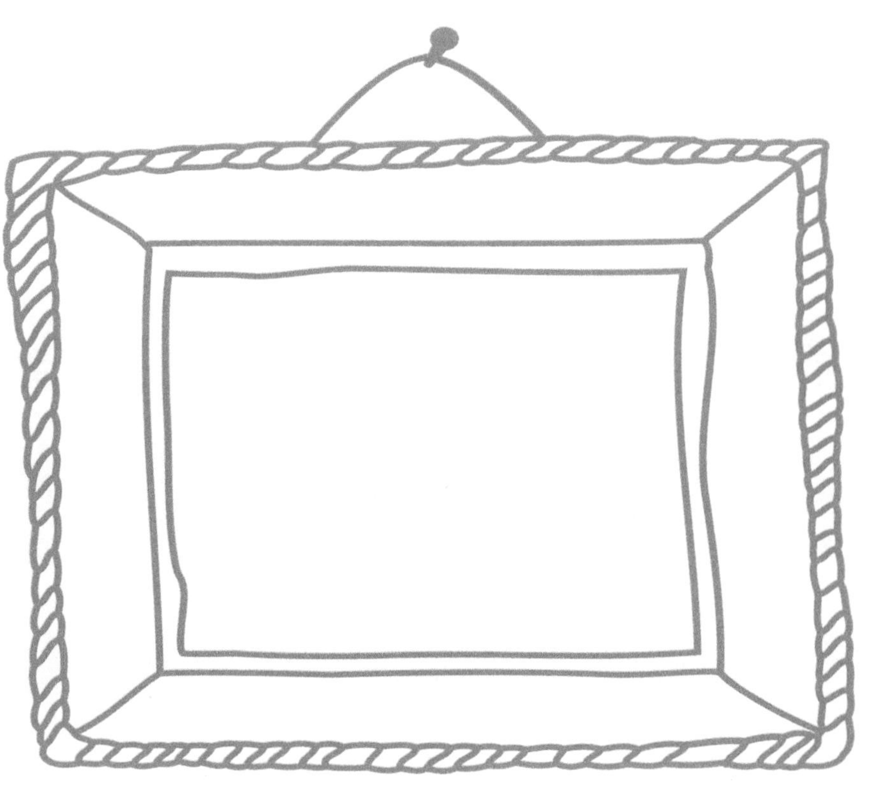

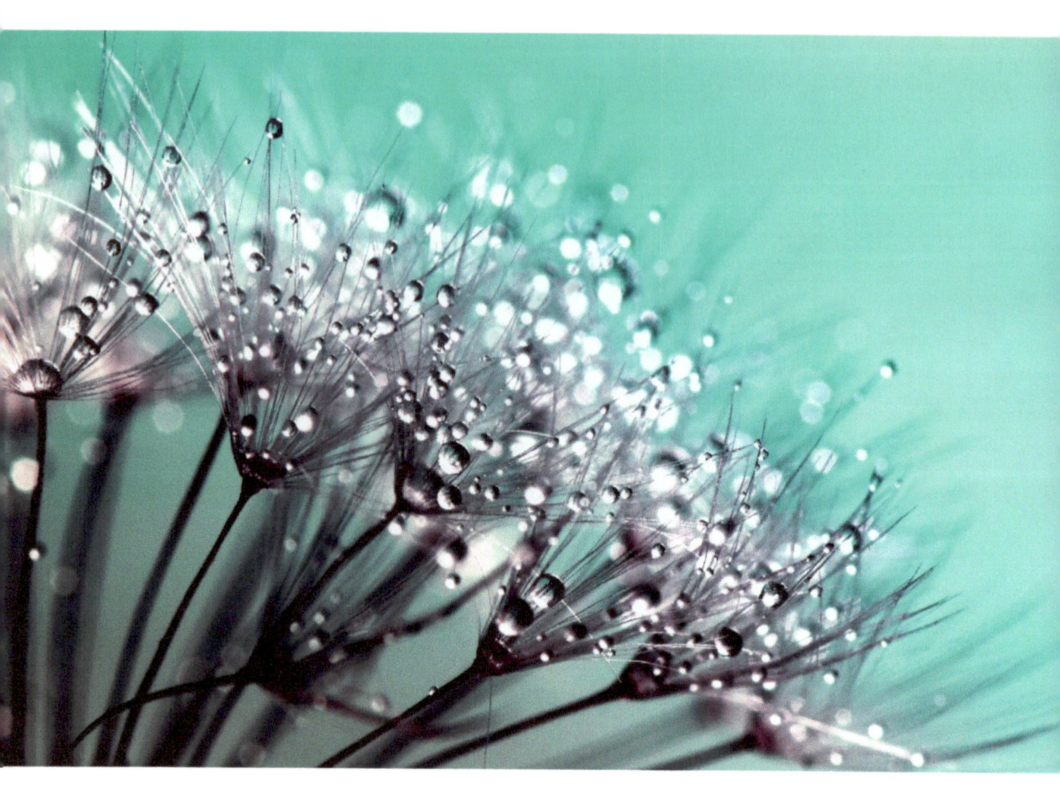

Focus on one element of the picture. Explain your thought process.

____

____

What calms you in this image?

____

____

What key feelings does this image make you think about?

____

____

Where in your own life calms and grounds you like this image?

____

____

Additional thought processes:

____

____

____

____

____

____

____

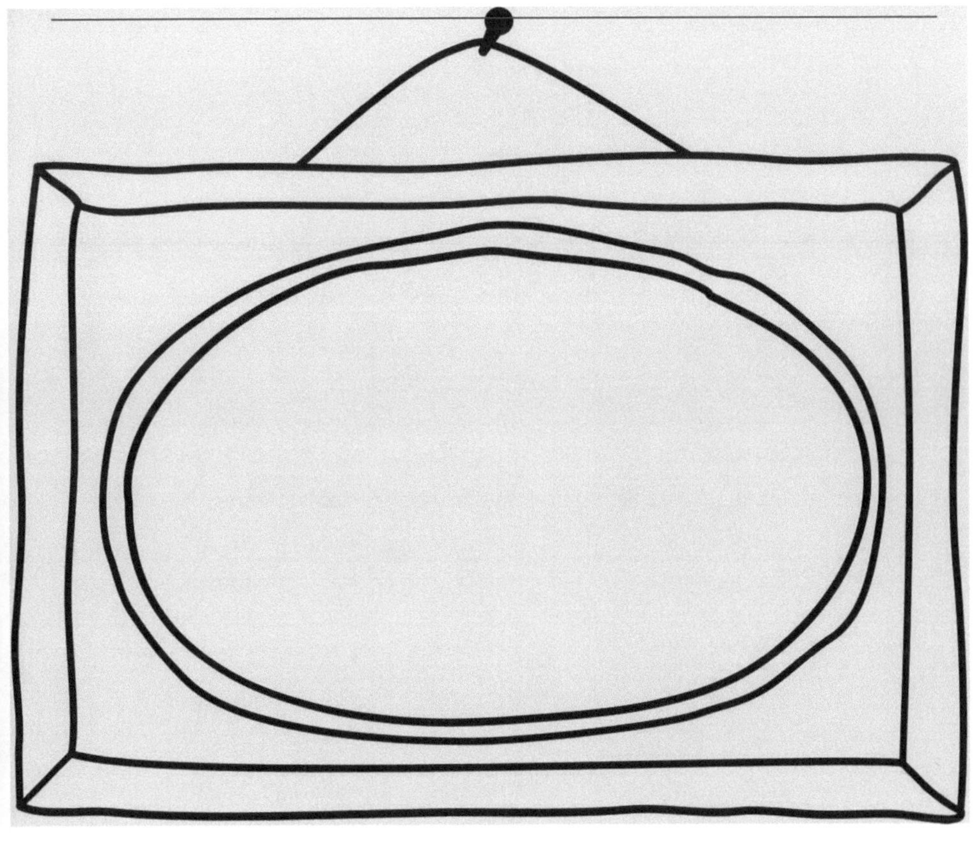

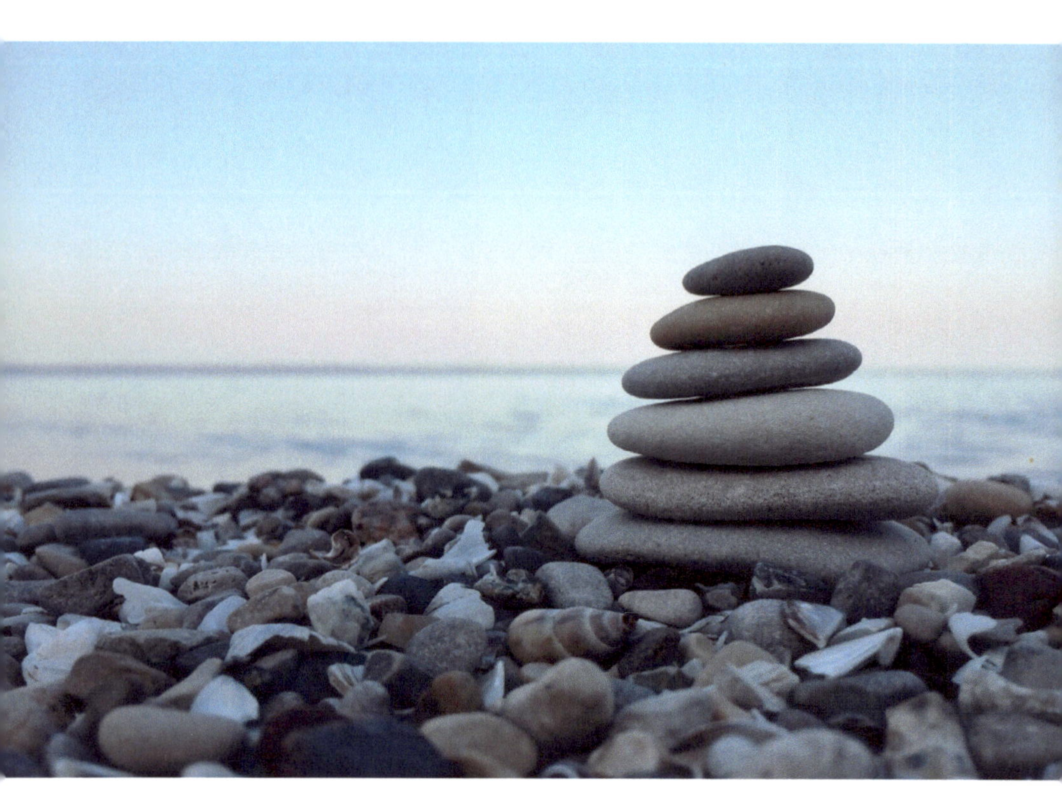

What is your main focus when you look at this image?

____

____

What does that focus remind you of?

____

____

Identify all of the elements of this image that appeal to you.

____

____

What music does this image make you think of?

____

____

If you have access, pop this music on now and just feel the 'music'.

Additional thought processes:

____

____

____

____

____

____

____

____

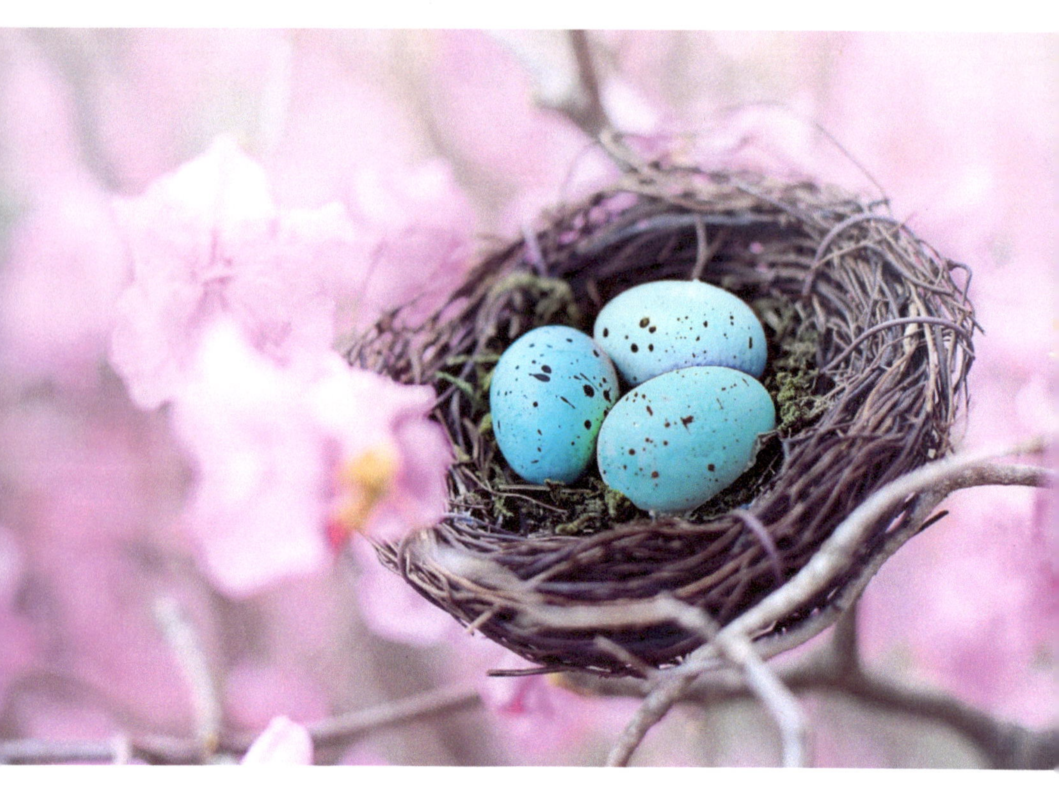

Where does this image place you?

____

____

Why did looking at the image place you where you suggested?

____

____

Focus on something from your memory when you placed yourself in this image. Explain your thought process.

____

____

With your though process linked to your placement,
explain the temperature evoked?

____

____

Additional thought processes:

____

____

____

____

____

____

____

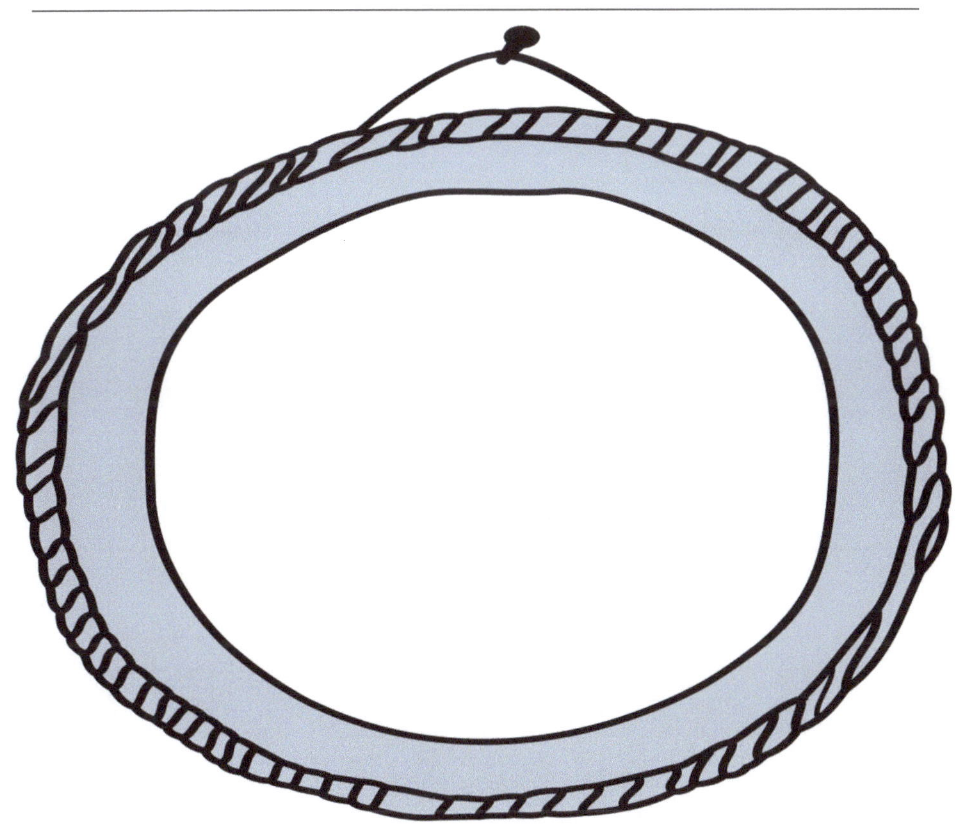

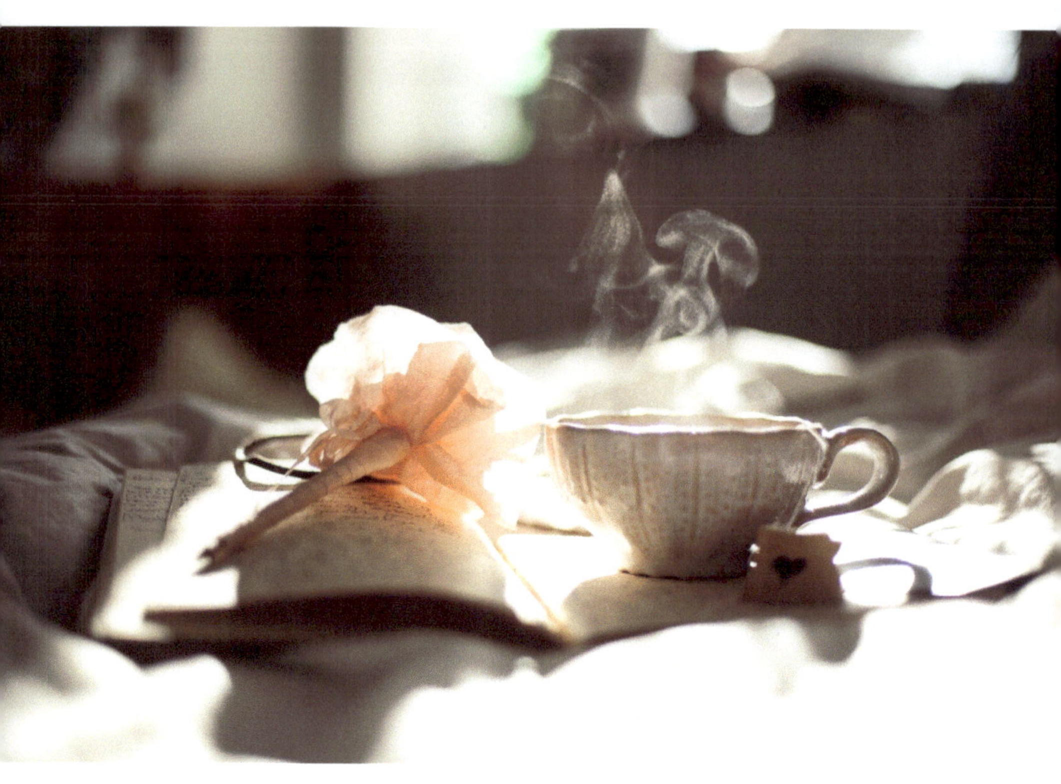

What does this image make you think of?
____
____

Think about your senses, what do you hear, feel, see, touch, smell?
____
____

Which sense is the strongest and why?
____
____

Explore that dominant sense and identify the thoughts related to it.

____

____

Additional thought processes:

____

____

____

____

____

____

____

____

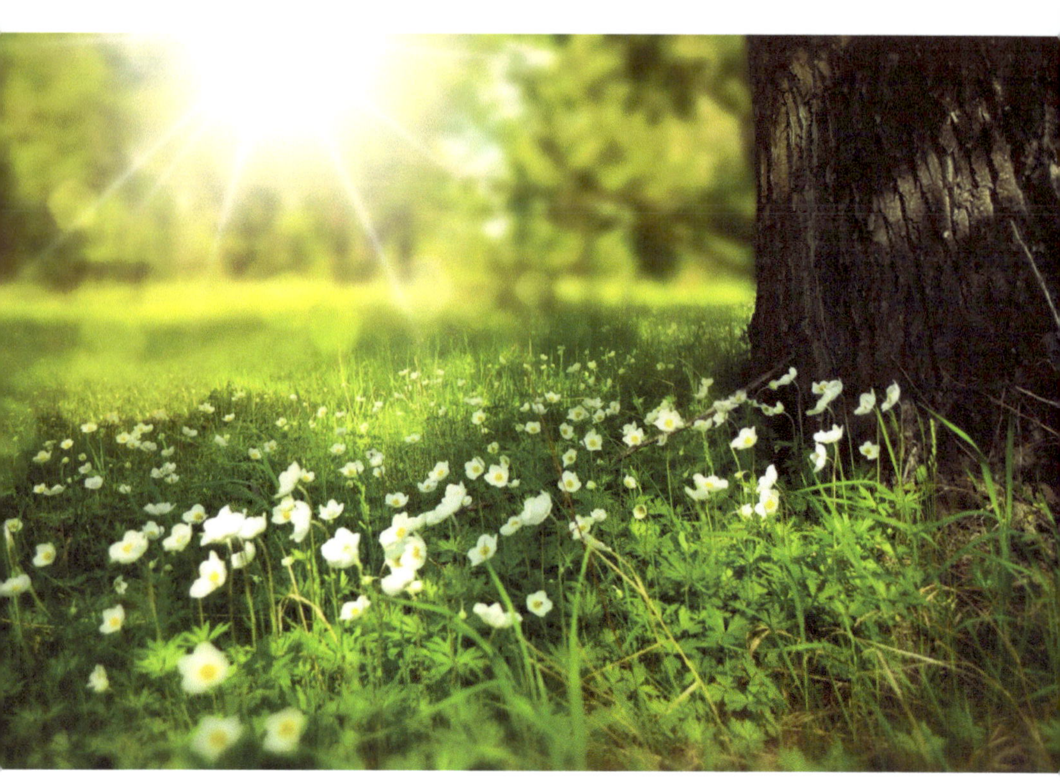

Place yourself in this image. Where are you?

____

____

Why did you choose this place?

____

____

Why do you think this image brought you to this place?

____

____

Think of a name that you can give this place so that
you can bring it back to you whenever you need to.

____

____

Additional thought processes:

____

____

____

____

____

____

____

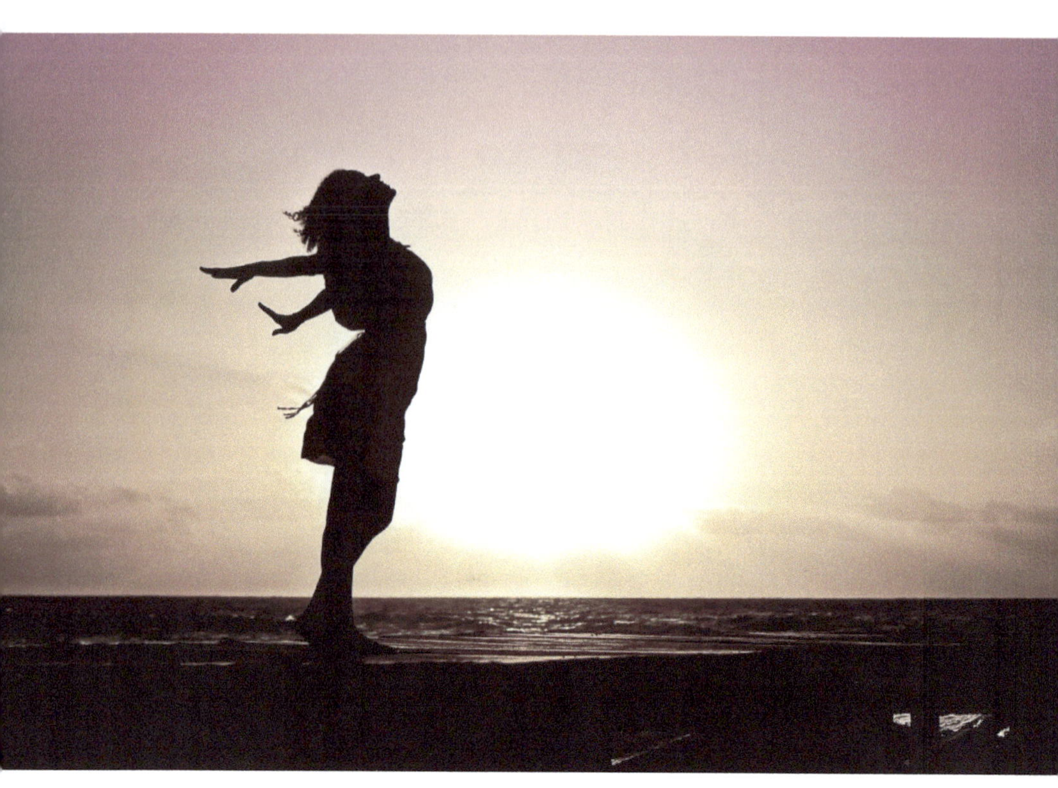

Place yourself in this image. Where are you looking out to?

____

____

How do you feel?

____

____

What do you hear?

____

____

Linger there a while and look around you, describe what you see and how you feel in more detail.

Now think of some of your own 'Safe Place
images' – you can draw, explain or print out images,
then explore your feeling, thoughts and emotions
linked to it.

1.

2.

3.

4.

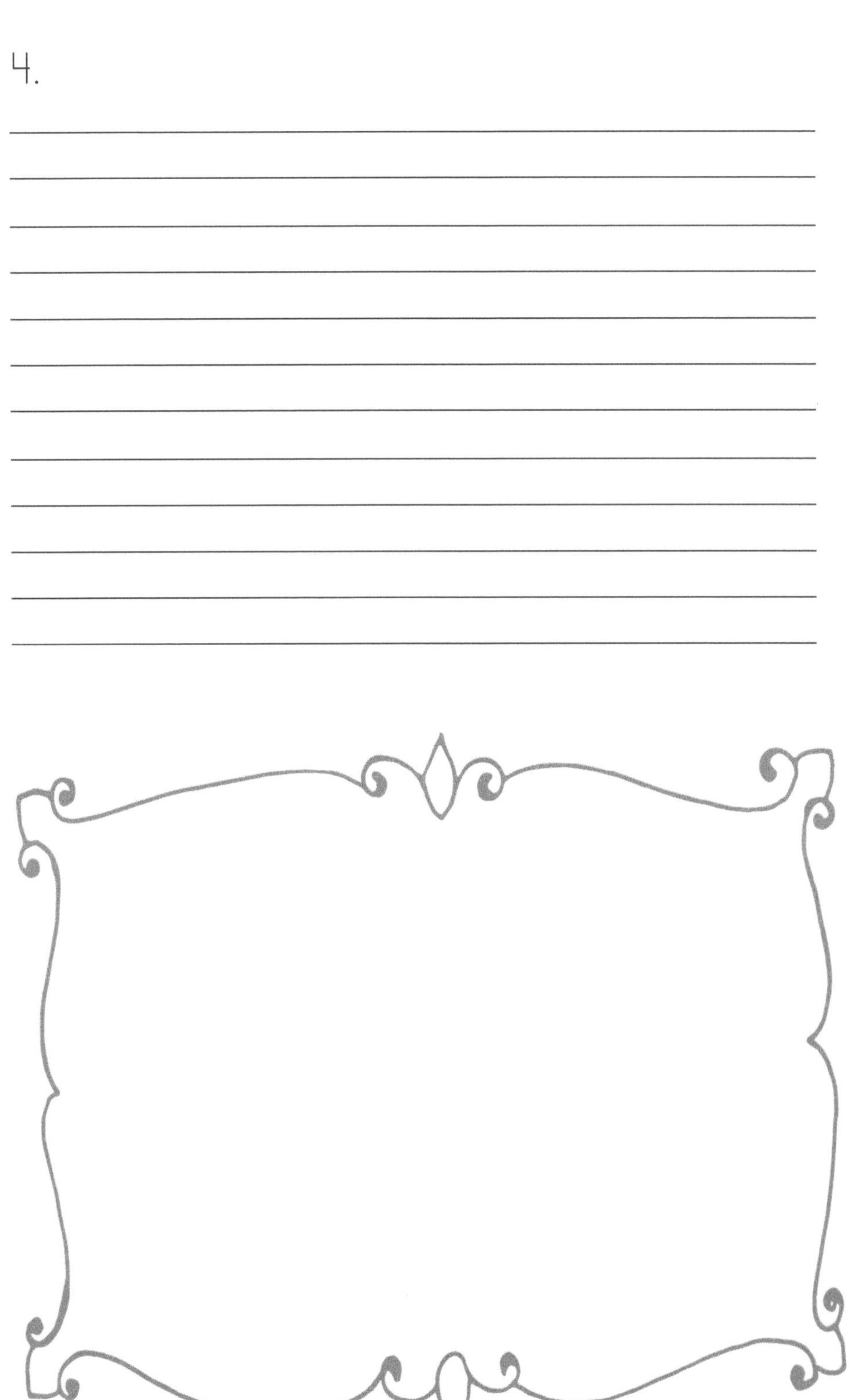

1.

2.

3.

4.

1.

2.

3.

4.

1.

2.

3.

4.

Appendix

'A wheel of emotions' to help identify emotions and support understanding how you are feeling.

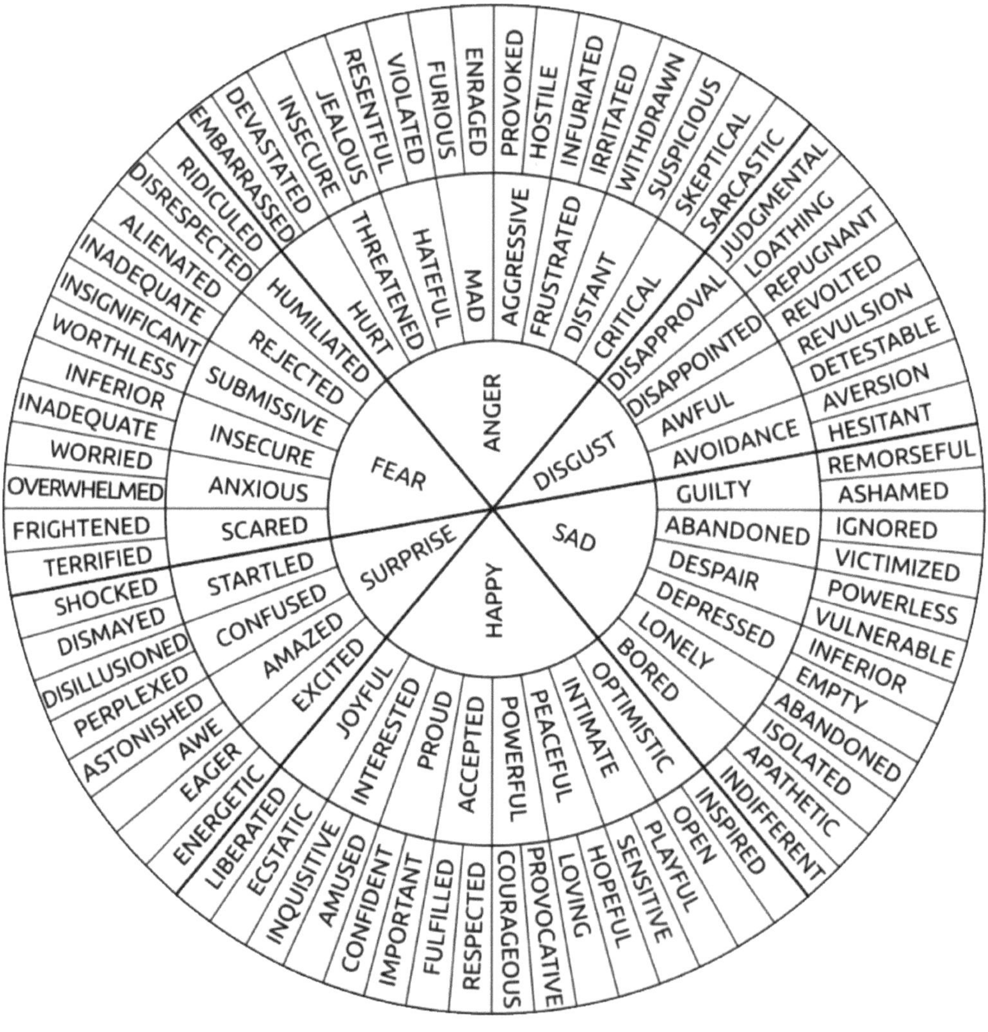

ANGER — FEAR — DISGUST — SAD — HAPPY — SURPRISE

ENRAGED, PROVOKED, HOSTILE, INFURIATED, IRRITATED, WITHDRAWN, SUSPICIOUS, SKEPTICAL, SARCASTIC, JUDGMENTAL, LOATHING, REPUGNANT, REVOLTED, REVULSION, DETESTABLE, AVERSION, HESITANT, REMORSEFUL, ASHAMED, IGNORED, VICTIMIZED, POWERLESS, VULNERABLE, INFERIOR, EMPTY, ABANDONED, ISOLATED, APATHETIC, INDIFFERENT, OPEN, INSPIRED, PLAYFUL, SENSITIVE, HOPEFUL, LOVING, PROVOCATIVE, COURAGEOUS, RESPECTED, FULFILLED, IMPORTANT, CONFIDENT, AMUSED, INQUISITIVE, ECSTATIC, LIBERATED, ENERGETIC, EAGER, AWE, ASTONISHED, PERPLEXED, DISILLUSIONED, DISMAYED, SHOCKED, TERRIFIED, FRIGHTENED, OVERWHELMED, WORRIED, INADEQUATE, INFERIOR, WORTHLESS, INSIGNIFICANT, INADEQUATE, ALIENATED, RIDICULED, DISRESPECTED, EMBARRASSED, DEVASTATED, INSECURE, JEALOUS, RESENTFUL, VIOLATED, FURIOUS, FURIOUS, MAD, AGGRESSIVE, FRUSTRATED, DISTANT, CRITICAL, DISAPPROVAL, DISAPPOINTED, AWFUL, AVOIDANCE, GUILTY, ABANDONED, DESPAIR, DEPRESSED, LONELY, BORED, OPTIMISTIC, INTIMATE, PEACEFUL, POWERFUL, ACCEPTED, PROUD, INTERESTED, JOYFUL, EXCITED, AMAZED, CONFUSED, STARTLED, SCARED, ANXIOUS, INSECURE, SUBMISSIVE, REJECTED, HUMILIATED, HURT, THREATENED, HATEFUL, MAD

HATEFUL, THREATENED, HURT, REJECTED, SUBMISSIVE, INSECURE, ANXIOUS, SCARED, STARTLED, CONFUSED, AMAZED, EXCITED, JOYFUL, INTERESTED, PROUD, ACCEPTED, POWERFUL, PEACEFUL, INTIMATE, OPTIMISTIC, HUMILIATED

www.ingramcontent.com/pod-product-compliance
Lightning Source LLC
Chambersburg PA
CBHW040316240726
48664CB00006B/1504